I0411491

Stairway To Heavenly Sleep

Your Step-By-Step Guide To Teaching
Your Baby To Sleep Through The Night

By

L. Christina O'Brien

1

Stairway To Heavenly Sleep

Is Dedicated To:

My four precious children:
Jayden, Justin, Katelyn and Jasmine.

Thank you all for letting me get some sleep.

Table Of Contents

Introduction

*O*ver the years, I've met quite a few mothers who were struggling with lack of sleep following the birth of their baby. In this book, I will be sharing the sleep method that I created to get my babies to sleep through the night, at a very young age.

At the time this book was written, I had four young children under the age of seven. Jayden, our oldest son, was sleeping through the night at eight weeks old. (By through the night, I mean eight consecutive hours without waking for milk). Our second son, Justin, was sleeping through the night at seven weeks old; Katelyn, our first daughter, was sleeping through the night at eight DAYS old, and all three were sleeping 12 consecutive hours without waking by 12 weeks old.

Once we had our second daughter, Jasmine, I was so busy with the other three children that I didn't follow my own sleep method as closely, and I paid for my mistake!

I soon realized I couldn't handle the night waking anymore, as I was getting too worn out looking after all four children on such little sleep. So I put my method into practice again and within a short period of time, we had another child who slept, often more than 12 consecutive hours, by six months of age.

In this easy-to-read book, I will show you exactly how my method works, step by step. I believe it can work for most babies, and in many situations. I understand you are tired! Whether you are pregnant and planning ahead, or if you are already a parent who has not had a good night's sleep for as long as you can remember, I am here to tell you, there IS HOPE! Keep reading and I believe my method will be a blessing to you and your kids! Soon, you will also be on your way to experiencing heavenly sleep!

Chapter 1

Sleep: One Of My Best Friends

"You better sleep now, while you can, since you probably won't get much sleep for the next 18 years!" Says the friendly stranger in the Walmart lineup with a smile. You bravely let out a nervous chuckle as you attempt to come up with a witty comment to continue the friendly conversation, but nothing comes to mind. She takes another glance at your now overdue, oversized, pregnant belly.

"When are you due?" She asks.

"Yesterday," you reply with anticipation. "I can hardly wait. It's my first child."

It's your turn in line. You put your purchases on the belt.

The friendly stranger looks at your box of newborn size diapers. "It's so hard to believe my kids once fit into those little things. They're all grown up now." She says.

"How many children do you have?" You ask her.

"I have five. Two boys and three girls. I haven't had a good night's sleep in 15 years. It was so hard...but now that they're all grown up, I can sleep again." She replies, trying to restore hope after she sees your reaction.

"Oh, it can't be that bad...can it?" You ask nervously.

"Well, you get used to the sleepless nights, but the overwhelming love you will have for your baby, will make it all worthwhile. Don't worry dear; you will be just fine." She says.

You put your bags into your cart. "Well, hopefully I'll be ok. You had five kids and you survived! I'm going to go to sleep when I get home while I still can!" You say with a smile.

"Good idea! And congratulations on your baby!" She calls out as you walk out of the store.

Wow, was she right? Is this possibly the last day you will ever sleep uninterrupted again?

The good news is, there IS a way to get sleep after your baby is born! I, personally, had suffered with sleep disorders my whole life. I have experienced what it was like to be tired for decades. I tried everything I could think of, including sleeping pills; but somehow, I was never able to get into a deep sleep. The insomnia I suffered with was so severe, that it would take me between six and

12 hours to fall asleep, every night. Some nights, I wouldn't fall asleep at all. I considered it to be a victory if I could fall asleep within three hours.

Throughout the years, my body was breaking down. I needed sleep. Sleep is one of our best friends! We just cannot function, to our greatest potential, without enough proper deep sleep. Everyone needs sleep and rest. Even God rested on the seventh day of creation:

By the seventh day, God had finished the work He had been doing;
So on the seventh day He rested from all His work.
−Genesis 2:2 NIV

When I found out that I was pregnant with our first child, I made the decision to stop taking my sleeping pills because I felt that it was better for the growing life inside of me. The insomnia, coupled with my anticipation of how my entire life was going to change, eight months from that day, made sleep even harder to come by.

I literally barely slept for the first five months of my pregnancy. I had to quit my job in the first month because I could no longer function without enough sleep. Six months into my pregnancy, I broke down. I started to pray more specific prayers than what I had been used to:

God, I am barely making it right now, as it is, with so little sleep. How am I supposed to be a mother and take care of someone else when I am already too tired to take care of myself? I can't do it. I just can't be a mother on no sleep. I need a miracle. I need you to do something Lord, or I won't be able to go on.

I would go as far as to say that I begged God, Jesus, and the Holy Spirit, on a daily basis, to intervene in my situation! Not much seemed to happen. I was already constantly exhausted, getting depressed, my body was physically weak, and I was losing hope. But I never lost faith.

I couldn't see how my situation could improve, especially when there was a baby coming into the mix that would probably cry half the night and wake me every hour. My patience was already worn thin through my exhaustion. How could I have patience for a baby? I couldn't see how it could change, but I had faith.

For we live by faith, not by sight.
−2 Corinthians 5:7 NIV

I prayed and I prayed and I prayed...*I just can't be a mother on such little sleep. Please help me Lord.* I prayed and prayed some more.

Pray continually, give thanks
in all circumstances.
−1 Thessalonians 5:17—18 NIV

When I was 38 weeks pregnant, our baby Jayden was born. After two days of hard labor, and barely a minute of sleep in over 60 hours, the labor ended in a cesarean section. I had three days in the hospital to enjoy my first precious times with my beautiful baby boy…It should have been a blissful time, except it turned out to be a sleepless nightmare!

I had only slept one and a half hours total in those three days! I was sent home on day three, feeling like a zombie, who was in terrible pain from just having had surgery, and was an emotional and hormonal wreck; and now I have this helpless little baby who is counting on me for everything, when I have nothing left to give.

I needed sleep. Without sleep, we can't recover. Our tank is empty. We are just running on fumes. Nobody can keep that up for too long! I kept on praying. I still had faith that God would come through for me. Then...it happened!

On day five, I was already ready to give up. 25 years of not sleeping well, a crying baby, and pain from the surgery had met the end of me. I gave up. I could no longer be a mother. I didn't have the strength in me. I told God that I needed help now or I just couldn't do it. Then, almost in the same thought, the Holy Spirit came upon me, and literally within one second, the answer on how to get my baby to sleep through the night, with details and steps, routines and time frames etc, was downloaded into my spirit instantly! Not only that, I was instantly healed of insomnia!!

How did I know I was healed right then? I don't know how I knew, I just knew. And then when I went to bed that night, I fell asleep! I can't even express how much of a miracle this was (and still is).

I went from waiting between six and 12 hours to fall asleep every night and still not experiencing deep sleep, to falling asleep in five to 30 minutes, and sleeping very well! So even though my baby was waking up several times throughout the night, for the first few weeks, I was sleeping better than I ever had; and because of this sleep method the Lord gave me, by the time Jayden was eight weeks old, I was sleeping all night long, and it was nothing short of heavenly sleep.

I want to share this gift of sleep that I received, with you.

Chapter 2

Setting The Stage
For A Good Night's Sleep

*E*very baby and every situation is different. There are exceptions to every rule, but by following my method, it is possible for full term babies under normal circumstances to sleep the corresponding number of hours to their age in weeks from age seven weeks to 12 weeks old.

For example, a seven week old baby can be expected to sleep seven consecutive hours at night, an eight week old baby, eight hours, etc. Some may sleep longer hours earlier, while others may sleep shorter hours later. I will write in average terms for what I know is possible, and so you have an idea of what you and your baby are aiming for.

The two most important things to keep in mind, while reading this book and implementing this method:

1. Your maternal or paternal instincts should be put above anything you read in this book.

2. If your baby was premature, you may need to feed more often than what I will outline in the daily schedules. Keep in mind, my schedule is written out for average situations and normal circumstances.

No matter what your situation may be, I am confident that you will find many, if not all of my tips very helpful. The more steps you follow, the more successful you will be.

Firstly, I don't believe babies are born either "good sleepers" or "bad sleepers." I believe that if the parents know how to teach their baby to sleep, then their baby will learn to be a good sleeper. Routine is the key! If you can create a plan and a routine and stick to it, your baby will figure it out, and sleep accordingly when you teach him it's time to sleep.

In the next chapter, you will find a chart that you can fill out to match what you want your lifestyle to look like. If you don't want your baby waking up at 6 a.m. on a Saturday morning, choose to teach him to sleep through past 6 a.m. on a Saturday morning. You can teach your baby to sleep and wake at whatever time of day you want him to. His schedule can easily be changed, if you need it to, when he is old enough to go to school.

The best time to plan your sleep schedule is actually BEFORE your baby is even born. If you already have a baby and a routine that just isn't working as well as you would like, we can change that as well. The earlier you plan it out, the sooner your baby will sleep through the night. If your baby is born into a set routine and continues with that same routine from birth, he will settle into his life of scheduled sleep fairly easily. (When I say fairly easily, I mean that we are aiming for 12 consecutive hours by 12 weeks old.)

Some things, we will be paying close attention to, in order to get your baby to learn how to sleep well:

1. Feeding schedule (This book is written in terms of breastfeeding, but if you are formula feeding, it works just the same)
2. Nap times
3. Bedtime routine
4. White noise
5. Music
6. Lighting
7. Swaddling
8. Sleeping arrangements

I will also be introducing you to what I call 'time blocks'. These blocks of time in the day are the time spacings between each activity that you will be filling out in your personalized chart, following my time blocks model.

OK! Let's get started!

Chapter 3

Planning Out Your Time Schedule
(Your Two-Year-Old Chart)

This chapter is all about forward thinking. Don't think about what you want your baby to do now yet. Think about how you want things to look when your baby is two years old.

At two years old, your baby should be sleeping 12 consecutive hours at night, and have a two to three-hour nap during the day. Let's just take a two-hour nap at age two as an example, just so you can fill out your chart, for now. You will use the times in the two-year-old chart as a model to fill in your times for your other charts.

You may already know what time you want your baby to sleep and wake. However, if you don't, here are a few things to consider:

1. Are you a morning person or a night person?
2. Do you want time to take showers in the mornings or before bed?
3. Do you like to sleep in or spend time alone in the mornings?
4. Do you prefer to go to bed early in the evenings?
5. Would you rather have your time away from the kids in the mornings or in the evenings?
6. What times are most convenient for you and you spouse to spend alone together?
7. Do you prefer to run your errands in the mornings, afternoons or evenings?
8. Are you a stay-at-home mom, or do you need your baby to sleep according to

your work schedule or his daycare schedule?

9. Who will be waking the baby for the day, and what time is convenient for them to stick to?

10. Who will be putting the child to bed for the night, and what time is convenient for them?

Some of these things may not seem important now, but trust me, if you plan it out, your life will be just a little bit easier, and you will be on the road to creating much needed time for yourself again. Not only will you be sleeping well, but you will also have time to do a few things that you want to do or that need to get done, and you will have time for showers!

The structure is so important for the whole family, and everyone will be happier for it. Sometimes, in the craziness of being a parent, we tend to forget about taking care of ourselves; but if you look after your own needs and take care of yourself, you will be stronger emotionally and physically to be the best parent you can be!

Instructions:

By the time your baby is two years old, we are aiming for his nap time to be four and a half hours after he wakes up, and he will wake from his nap two hours later, which means he will wake from his nap five and a half hours before he goes to bed for the night based on a 12-hour night sleep.

For example, if you want your child to go to bed at 9 p.m., and wake up at 9 a.m. when he is two years old, (you can change it for school aged children later on.) his nap time will be from 1:30 p.m. to 3:30 p.m., so you will fill in your chart as such:

2 Year Chart

	9:00 AM	Wake up for the day
Add 4.5 Hours	1:30 PM	Put down for a nap
Add 2 Hours	3:30 PM	Wake up from nap
Add 5 Hours	8:30 PM	Start bedtime routine
Add Half an Hour	9:00 PM	Say goodnight!

You will be using the same charts for the weekdays and the weekends.

Another example, if you want your child's sleep and wake times to be 7 a.m. and 7 p.m., his nap time will be from 11:30 a.m., to 1:30 p.m.

If you work the night shift and if an 11:30 a.m. wake up time and 11:30 p.m. bedtime works better for you, then make that your routine. In this case, your child should nap from 4 p.m. to 6 p.m.

Yes, you can teach them to sleep the hours that work for you!

Now for your first portion of homework, fill out your own chart with the times you envision your two-year-old to be sleeping and napping, following my time blocks model:

		2 Year Chart
		Wake up for the day
Add 4.5 Hours		Put down for a nap
Add 2 Hours		Wake up from nap
Add 5 Hours		Start bedtime routine
Add Half an Hour		Say goodnight!

Good work! That looks good to me. We can definitely work with this.

Chapter 4

Understanding And Tricking
Your Newborn

So, your baby is due any day now. You are double-checking that you have everything you need packed for the hospital. Diapers: Check. Wipes: Check. Sleepers: Check. Hats and socks for baby: Check...and the list goes on.

But did you pack what you will need to start teaching your newborn baby to sleep? Starting from birth is best! I would like you to bring a music player with kids' lullabies or soothing music that you can see yourself using for quite a while.

When babies are born, they naturally have their days and nights reversed. Almost every baby will seem to sleep all day, then when you finally get to lie down after a long day, your baby is wide awake! It's not just your baby! This is normal! Your baby doesn't just wake up when you want to lie down, he probably also cries for you until you get up. Lovely. Why does this happen?

Well, put yourself in your baby's shoes for a moment...or his booties for that matter. You're used to being in the womb. The most comforting place ever. You're all cuddled up. When mommy is awake, walking and talking, you are being rocked to sleep in the womb by her movements, and her comforting voice is just the peace you need for sweet sleep. But...when she lies down for bed, the rocking stops and you no longer hear the comforting sounds that rocked you to sleep during the day.

Ok, now put your own shoes back on. Did you ever notice that while you were pregnant, you didn't seem to feel the baby's movements much while you were awake and walking around, but as soon as you try to sleep is when your baby thinks its time to play soccer with your ribs and your bladder?

Taking note that this is the case, is your first step toward eventually getting your own sleep. You need to teach your baby to sleep during the hours that you want him to, but he only wants to sleep during the daytime, so my first major tip for a newborn baby is:

During the night, in the first week or two, you need to trick your baby into thinking the night is day, because if he thinks it's daytime, he will sleep better.

Think of what he likes during the day that he associates with sleeping. Noise, comforting familiar voices, and light. Yes, babies can see light while they are in the womb. Also, after birth, they sleep well when they are being held.

While it's one of the most wonderful feelings to have your baby fall asleep in your arms, you won't be able to get your own sleep, if your baby can ONLY sleep when he is in your arms.

Don't worry; this sleep method will still allow you to experience your baby sleeping in your arms; but we will teach him to sleep in his own bassinet or crib when it's time for you to sleep, or when it's time for what I call his "official" naps and sleeps.

First, I will talk about how to trick your baby into believing it is daytime when it is actually nighttime. Then we will go over the newborn schedule, in the next chapter, which will include all feeding times to prepare your baby to sleep that heavenly eight-hour stretch by eight weeks old.

Instructions:

So I mentioned noise, comforting familiar voices, light, and being held, as the main factors why newborns have their days and nights reversed.

Noise:

The noise method comes in two steps: **The first is white noise. Put a fan in the room your baby will be sleeping in.** Aim it away from him of course. This will help to block out noises he would otherwise hear during his official sleep times. I use the white noise method indefinitely, every single night. That way when your baby is napping, or sleeping at night, before you go to bed, you won't have to tiptoe around, afraid to wake up your baby, and the continuous sound helps them sleep better as well.

The second part, of the noise method, is to use nice soft music. In the first week or two, I want you to **put the music on repeat so it stays on continuously, all night long**, and set the volume to a level you might use when you have the television on during the day. If you tend to have a rather loud lifestyle with your family, keep your baby's music on loud. If you have a quieter family, you can lower the volume.

The main idea is you want your baby to think it's daytime, for the time being, and the comforting music will replace the comforting sounds he slept to in the womb during the day. Always use the same music, because within two months, he will associate the particular songs to knowing when it's time to sleep.

Light:

You will need to get blackout curtains or blinds to block out ALL the sunlight from your baby's room. If blackout curtains or blinds are not in your budget, you can tape tin foil to your window. (Do not use black garbage bags! The heat from the sun's reflection will crack your window panes.) This is a very important step toward having your baby sleep the hours that you want him to.

Babies and kids tend to wake up with the sunlight; and when it comes to time changes, and the sunrise and sunsets being at totally different hours during different seasons, your child's sleep will be all over the place; and I can assure you, he will end up waking you at 6 a.m. because the sun told him to. If your baby's room is as dark as possible, he will learn to sleep according to the time charts that <u>you</u> fill out. In the first week or two however, even though the sunlight is blocked out, I want you to **keep the light in the room on all night** to help mimic the daytime.

Being Held:

The last way you can trick your baby to sleep is what I call "the fake arms wrap". Your baby will want you to hold him to go to sleep, but in the long run, this is just not realistic if your ultimate goal is to put him down to sleep so that you can go to your own bed and sleep.

Keeping your long-term goals in mind is very important, and requires establishing good sleeping habits now. It is much harder to change your baby's habits later, than it is to start him with your goal habits from day one.

So how do you trick your baby into thinking someone is holding him when he's not being held? Get him in a good swaddle where he can't get his arms out. Lie him down in his bassinet or crib, then use a second long blanket, place it on top of him so the top of the blanket is at his shoulders and roll or bunch the sides up close to him so he is tucked in between two "arm-sized" rolls. And there you have it. Fake arms. Just make sure the room is not too warm when you do this.

Depending on which hours you chose, in your two-year-old chart, and what time of day your baby was born, you could have your baby's night and day reversal switched back to normal in about two weeks, on average. Do not be discouraged if it takes longer. He will get it soon, if you stick to the schedule as closely as possible.

Chapter 5

Establishing A Bedtime Routine

I believe that establishing a bedtime routine is very important, even as early as day one. Your baby will quickly start to recognize the series of events in your bedtime routine, and associate them with sleep. It is important that the routine is as similar as possible every night. You may want to change it slightly, as your baby gets older, to be age appropriate, but you will still be generally doing the same types of things.

For example, before one year of age, your bedtime routine will include milk feedings; but after that, it may or may not, depending on what you choose to do. Also, you may not want to read bedtime stories to your newborn, but you might want to a few months from now. You decide!

Your bedtime routine can include different types of signals to your baby. The time on the clock is not as important to your baby as the audio and visual routine. The routine signals can be small (like going upstairs, turning on a lamp, closing curtains, etc.) mixed with larger signals (bath time, listening to music together, reading stories, watching TV, etc.). Within a few weeks, when you start your bedtime routine with your baby, he will already be making a connection between the routine and knowing that this signals bedtime.

The routine you choose should be anywhere between 15 and 45 minutes. I use a 30-minute bedtime routine in my schedule to make the charts a little easier for you to fill out and to follow.

Babies find routine very comforting. When they know what to expect, they feel safer. I even go as far as saying the same sentences every night to my kids and my baby as I'm closing their doors for the night. I've been playing the same songs to them, and saying the same goodnight sentences for years, and they never get tired of them:

"Goodnight! Sleep Tight. See you in the morning. You're so special, I love you!" is what you will hear in my household four times per night. In fact, this method is so effective, that when they hear a song, come on the Christian radio station in the van, that I put on for them at bedtime, they sometimes fall asleep because they associate those particular songs with sleeping!

Your next item of homework is to think, for a few moments, about what you would want to create as your bedtime routine. Consider what will work for the family, and try to pick something that you can do every night, if possible. Jot down some notes on a separate sheet of paper, if you wish. It may help to have it written down as you get used to using this sleep method.

Babies tend to feel extra sleepy after a nice warm bath, but bathing a newborn every day can dry out their skin, so if you choose bath time, as part of your nightly routine, you might want to consider massaging some lotion onto their skin. Baby massage is also very calming for babies. They love it; it helps you and your baby bond, and it also provides health benefits! Lavender baby soaps in their bath do work to soothe them during bath time as well.

Another thing to keep in mind, is that a warm bath can make them TOO sleepy to feed properly before you try to put them to bed for the night; which means they will wake up sooner for another feeding. If you want to use bath time, as a means to help your baby sleep, don't dress him right away afterwards, but do keep him warm. Not dressing him right away should keep him awake enough to feed well before bed.

It is also important that your baby's pajamas are the same type of pajamas every night until at least 18 months of age. Warm sleepers are my favorite choice. If you don't have air conditioning, you may want to do diaper shirts (onesies) during the summer, and sleepers during the winter, for example. Believe it or not, they will even associate the type of outfit with bedtime. I see it happen all the time. Newborns also tend to sleep better when they wear hats to keep them warm and cozy.

When deciding which type of outfit to use as your baby's pajamas, you will also want to consider what I call the "burrito wrap" method so your baby doesn't get too hot at night. Of all the things I have mentioned thus far in this book, I would have to say that the "burrito wrap" is the technique that worked the best for me. You will be doing this wrap, right before you place them into their crib. If I wrap them in a regular swaddle, they just don't seem to sleep as long! (The "burrito wrap" also works wonders as the base for the "fake arms wrap" that I described earlier.)

What is the "burrito wrap?" Well, it's actually just like it sounds. Spread a rectangular blanket (or towel) onto a bed, near where your baby will be sleeping. If there's no bed nearby, you can "burrito wrap" him right in the crib, or on the floor as a last resort if you don't have a soft place where you can wrap him every night. Place your baby on the left side of the blanket or towel with his shoulders flush with the top edge of the blanket. Make sure his arms are by his side, and literally roll him up like a sausage. You will need to hold the blanket snug during the first turn so they end up being nice and snug as a bug in a rug.

What size blanket or towel should you use? Something long enough to make two or three full turns is ideal. It also helps them stay snug for longer if the end of the blanket ends up under them when you put them down so their body weight keeps the burrito closed. You don't want them to be able to get their arms out at the newborn stage or they will keep waking up.

If you start with the "burrito wrap" from day one, your baby will love it. Being tight and snug reminds them of being in the womb, which to them, at this point in their lives, was the best place in the world. Have your burrito blanket laid out and ready every night, before you nurse, so you are ready to wrap him when he falls asleep.

Don't forget to make bedtime a happy, fun, and loving experience! Lots of hugs, kisses and cuddles will go a long way to eventually having an older child who actually enjoys going to bed.

Quick Summary:

Lighting: Block out the sun with curtains or blinds, and leave the bedroom light ON in the first week or two to trick your baby into thinking that night is day.

White Noise: Keep a fan running, during official nap time and night sleep, to block out different noises that may disturb your baby, and to have the constant sound going which lulls them into a deeper sleep.

Music: Choose soothing music that you will continue to play nightly for your baby, so that he will associate it with bedtime, and leave it ON all night on repeat, in the first week or two (at a daytime noise level) while you are working on reversing their days to nights.

Bedtime Routine: Choose a routine that you can do every night to help your baby associate your actions with bedtime.

Swaddling: Practice the "burrito wrap" that you will put your baby in, for every official nap time and night sleep.

"Fake Arms Wrap:" For babies who don't seem to want to sleep, unless they are in mommy or daddy's arms.

Two-Year-Old Schedule Plan: You've established when you want your baby to nap and sleep when he is two years old.

In the next chapter, we will go over the detailed newborn schedule you can follow, that will eventually match up to your two-year-old planned schedule.

Chapter 6

Newborn Scheduling
And Nursing Tips

*C*ongratulations! You just had your baby. I hope the delivery went well for you. I'm guessing the nurses are telling you to feed your baby every three hours. While that is good advice, it's not optimal for getting your baby to sleep through the night very early, and, let's face it, you're very tired, and sleep has suddenly become more important to you than eating or showering.

Think about this: If a newborn needs to have between eight and 10 feedings in a 24-hour period for healthy weight gain, and if you are feeding every three hours around the clock, you will not get anything longer than a two and a half hour stretch of sleep at night considering the average baby who is nursing will feed for approximately 30 to 45 minutes per feeding at this stage...and that's if you fall asleep right away!

With this method, we are aiming for you to have a four and a half to five-hour stretch of sleep from day one. Yes, it is possible. It is more work during the day, and you may feel like all you ever do is feed your baby, but it will be worth it, if we can get him to sleep five hours for you right off the bat so you can be more rested. I am on your side. I have been there many times.

Your newborn schedule will have you feeding every two hours, for most of the day, with the exception of a three-hour nap near the middle of the day. I will be using the same 9 a.m. – 9 p.m. example throughout this book.

I actually like to work backwards. Instead of trying to put your baby to bed at 9 p.m. at this age, I suggest working it out so that they have their longest stretch of sleep before wake-up time. For example, we are immediately aiming for a five-hour stretch of sleep right after birth, so put your baby down for his night sleep at 4 a.m. (or line 12 from your newborn chart that you will fill out in chapter 7) to aim to have him wake up by 9 a.m. (or line 1 from your chart), and hopefully not before. Don't worry, you won't be doing this for too long. This is just the starting point.

Follow this same schedule every single day, until your baby really gets it. Hopefully, this will happen somewhere between week three and week five. If you are putting your baby to bed, for the night, at 4 a.m. (or line 12) but you find he is still in a deep sleep by 9 a.m. (line 1), he is ready to give you a sleep stretch longer than five hours. This is when you can start to consider putting him to sleep for the night at 3:30 a.m. (or half an hour before the time you will write on line 12 in your chart). If he wakes up before 9 a.m., continue this 3:30 a.m. bedtime routine until he is still asleep at 9 a.m. and it's you that has to wake him before he wakes on his own.

Once he has had several nights like this where you have to wake your baby at wake up time, it's time to move up bedtime again to 3 a.m. (or one hour before line 12 in your chart) until he is still asleep at 9 a.m. This will happen at different stages for each baby; but don't forget, we are aiming for eight consecutive hours, without waking for milk by eight weeks old, so there's still time.

Newborns sleep almost all the time (except when you want to sleep, it seems). They can sleep an average of 20 hours per day. This is why, introducing your baby to what I call "official naps/sleep" and "unofficial naps/sleep," as early as possible, is key to having him recognize when you will actually WANT him to sleep, when he gets a little bit older.

What do I mean by "official" and "unofficial sleep?"

Official Sleep: This is the scheduled nap time and sleep time, where you close the curtains to block out the sun, turn the lights on, and play the music on repeat (for the first two weeks), turn on the fan for white noise, give him his last feeding, then wrap him up with the "burrito wrap" and put him down to sleep in his crib or bassinet (alone preferably so you both can sleep more soundly).

Unofficial Sleep: This is all the other times of the day your baby falls asleep that are not official nap or sleep times. Your baby might fall asleep in your arms, during a car ride, cuddled with you in your bed while you try to doze during the day, in his swing, in his carrier, etc.

Try to keep his official nap in the same location every time, as long as you are home for nap time. He will quickly start to recognize that this is the place he is expected to have a longer sleep.

In the first two weeks, you need to try **to keep your baby awake for about half an hour before his official nap time, and**

official bedtime. This will help him sleep the right amounts of time to work with the schedule. With this in mind, you can still have naps or go to bed when he sleeps, just make sure you set an alarm to wake up in time for the scheduled feedings to stay on track. Just be sure to remember to try to keep him awake for that half-hour before the official sleeps to help him learn the routine.

Make sure, as much as possible, that your baby is having good feedings at every feeding time. This can be a challenge, because almost all newborns will fall asleep at every feeding. A baby who is drinking colostrum (the first milk that appears from the breast) needs to feed for about 45 minutes per feeding; (about 20 minutes from each breast).

Feeding from both sides will encourage your milk to come in faster, and encourage a higher volume of milk. The milk will appear somewhere around day two or three for a baby born vaginally, and somewhere between day three and five for babies born via cesarean section. If you have any concerns about your milk production, speak to your doctor, nurse, midwife, or lactation consultant.

Breast milk is the best option for babies. 99% of mothers are able to produce enough milk to nurse their babies exclusively if their babies get a good latch, nurse effectively, and the mother has adequate nutrition.

So how do you give your baby a productive feeding when all he wants to do is sleep? It is important, for your baby's health and weight gain, to do your best to wake him when it's time for a feeding, and to try to keep him awake while he is feeding. If you let him sleep whenever he wants, and let him wake up whenever he wants, it will be hard to get that glorious five-hour stretch of sleep at night that you are already longing for, and he may not get enough milk if he sleeps too long during the day. You are the boss, you tell your baby when it's time to wake up, eat and go to sleep, and he will catch on.

Here are some tips to try to keep your baby awake during feedings:

1. Tickle his jawbone to encourage swallowing.
2. Move his arms up and down.
3. Tickle those cute little toes.
4. Massage his feet.
5. Do the bicycle motion with his legs.
6. Take him off the breast, then put him back on again.
7. Change his position several times.
8. Put him down.
9. Take his clothes off, to cool him down. ("You're just too warm and cozy mommy!")
10. Change his diaper then try to feed him again.

Try everything you can think of, for at least 20–30 minutes, when your schedule says that it's time for a feeding. If all else fails, and he just won't stay awake but you feel he hasn't eaten enough, let him sleep for half an hour and try the waking methods again. If you feel he may have eaten enough, refer back to your schedule and just try again at the next feeding time. Use your instincts.

It can be difficult to get a newborn to comply with a set schedule like this one. If it just doesn't seem to be working and you're having trouble getting your baby to feed at your scheduled times, don't get discouraged. Remember, it is something we are aiming for to create structure for the long term. If it doesn't work today, try the same thing again tomorrow!

Great is His faithfulness; His mercies begin afresh each morning.
–Lamentations 3:23 NLT

Chapter 7

Your Newborn Schedule

*H*ere is more homework for you. Unlike most homework you got in elementary and high school, this homework will really benefit your life. Ha ha. Hey, you just had a baby, you deserve a little laugh.

So to fill out your newborn schedule, start with the wake up time from your two-year-old chart and write it down on line 1 of your newborn chart. Add the specified amount of hours from the second column to help you fill in the time column. See the 9 a.m. – 9 p.m. newborn example schedule below to help you out.

		Newborn Schedule	
Line 1	Use wake up time from 2 year chart	9 AM	Wake up for the day and Feed baby right away
2	Add 2 hours	11 AM	Feed Baby
3	Add 2 hours	1 PM	Feed Baby until he falls asleep
4	Add half an hour	1:30 PM	**Official Nap Time!**
5	Add 3 hours	4:30 PM	Wake baby up from nap and feed right away
6	Add 2 hours	6:30 PM	Feed baby
7	Add 2 hours	8:30 PM	Feed baby
8	Add 2 hours	10:30 PM	Feed baby
9	Add 2 hours	12:30 AM	Feed Baby
10	Add 2 hours	2:30 AM	Start bedtime routine and feed baby again
11	Add 1 hour	3:30 AM	Feed baby until he falls asleep for the night
12	Add half an hour	4 AM	**Official Sleep.** Say goodnight!
13	Add 5 hours	9 AM	Wake baby up for the day and feed.

Now here is your chart to fill out:

Newborn Schedule			
Line 1	Use wake up time from 2 year chart		Wake up for the day and Feed baby right away
2	Add 2 hours		Feed Baby
3	Add 2 hours		Feed Baby until he falls asleep
4	Add half an hour		**Official Nap Time!**
5	Add 3 hours		Wake baby up from nap and feed right away
6	Add 2 hours		Feed baby
7	Add 2 hours		Feed baby
8	Add 2 hours		Feed baby
9	Add 2 hours		Feed Baby
10	Add 2 hours		Start bedtime routine and feed baby again
11	Add 1 hour		Feed baby until he falls asleep for the night
12	Add half an hour		**Official Sleep.** Say goodnight!
13	Add 5 hours		Wake baby up for the day and feed.

Close to bedtime (starting at line 10), you will always want to do what we call cluster feedings. This is squeezing the last couple of feedings closer together, before the longest stretch of night sleep. If you are nursing, try to keep your baby awake long enough to feed from both sides twice, for his very last feed of the night. Aim to put him down, for the night, at the time you will enter in line 12 of your chart. This helps their tummies to be nice and full to help them sleep for longer stretches of time.

You should also try to sleep, when the baby sleeps, no matter what time of day it is at this stage. However, I suggest setting an alarm to make sure your baby is awake when you want him to be, and feeding when you want him to be.

Suggested order of steps for the last feed of the night:

Start by getting the room ready. Turn on the lights and put the music on repeat (just for the first week or two), turn on the white noise fan and close the curtains. If you start his feeding by undressing him, that should wake him enough to feed well. Start the feeding. If he dozes, change his diaper. If he dozes off again, dress him for the night. Just do things to keep stirring him. The burrito wrap should be attempted last, right before he goes in his crib. (Make sure you have laid out your blanket ahead of time in preparation for wrapping him up). Continue feeding until he seems fully asleep. (Later we will aim to have him fall asleep on his own, but for now, he can fall asleep by the end of the feeding).

Once he seems "out like a light," now is the time to wrap him. If the wrapping process has caused him to stir too much, nurse again until he falls asleep. Then place him down all wrapped up. If he doesn't like to be put down, try the "fake arms wrap" with a second blanket, described in chapter 4.

If your baby wakes up during his attempted five-hour stretch of sleep, do not talk to him, and do not change his diaper if it is just wet. Rewrap him and give him a quick feed while he is wrapped, burp him and place him down again quietly, gently

and softly. Not talking to him or changing his diaper will help him to stay in sleep mode. If he is stimulated and rewarded by conversation and extra actions from you, he will be wide awake again.

My recommended times for running errands, at this stage, is either between 10 a.m. and home by 12:30 p.m. (one hour after line 1, and half an hour before line 3), OR from 5 p.m. and home by 8 p.m. (half an hour after line 5, and half an hour before line 7).

If you must be out all day, try to work it out so that your baby has somewhere to sleep for his official nap time, to keep with the schedule as much as possible. If you are at someone's house, for example, and you know you can put your baby for a nap on someone's bed, be sure to bring your "burrito" blanket with you so you can wrap him, and he will still be somewhat familiar with the process until you can nap him at home again.

If you can't place him down to sleep, allow him to sleep in his car seat or stroller, for the three-hour time allotted for his official nap, if he will sleep that long. Just be sure to watch the time and wake him to feed as close to the planned time as possible.

You do not need to worry about how often he falls asleep, in the first two weeks. Just remember to try to keep your baby awake for a good half-hour before his official nap and sleep times. Soon, he will fall into a pattern of three scheduled naps a day.

If he doesn't seem tired enough for his official sleeps, consider keeping him awake for 45 minutes to an hour before his scheduled sleeps. Some of this depends on your individual baby. Trial and error, over time, will go a long way as well.

Chapter 8

Weeks 2 Through 4

*I*f you feel that your baby is doing reasonably well with sleeping, while you still have the lights and music on all night, to trick him into thinking your night is his day, it is time to start thinking of turning, what he thinks is still day into a new meaning of night.

So what is the next step in turning his days and nights around?

Music: Continue to keep the music on repeat all night long, but ever so gradually, turn the volume down in small increments. I would suggest turning it down slightly, once a week, until the music is at a nice quiet level. Eventually, you can take it off repeat and just have the music play through once, and see if he continues to sleep when it is quiet (with the exception of the white noise that is ideally always on). When you decide to do this, can be at your discretion, all the while taking your baby's cues as clues.

If he starts waking again at night when the music stops, put it back on repeat for another week and try again. The gradual change will help him adjust along the way.

Lighting: It's the same idea here as with the music. Gradually turn down the lights, once a week, until you have reached the lighting of a small night-light, so you can see what you're doing when you need to go in for night feedings. You do not want to walk into pitch-black darkness and turn on a light to feed your baby; you will just wake him up more. If you have a dimmer switch on the light where the baby is sleeping, it makes this process easier. If you don't, get creative! Change the light bulbs in lamps to lower wattage every week, or plug in smaller lamps. A sudden change in the lighting can cause him to not sleep his five-hour night increment. If you have trouble, put the original lighting, that you have been using, back on, until he is sleeping better again.

At this point, is if he has mastered his five-hour stretch of sleep, you can start trying to put him to bed earlier, by half-hour increments, until he has mastered each step, as I had described in chapter 6.

Also, around weeks two and three, he may need to be kept awake for about one hour, before his official naps and official night sleeps. By week four, he needs about one and a half hours of wake time before his official naps and sleeps for optimal sleep.

Chapter 9

Weeks 5 through 7

*T*he schedule here will change a little now. By age five to seven weeks old, your baby will need to be kept awake for about two hours before his official naps and sleep times, if possible, so that he is tired enough to sleep well, when you want him to; but you can still let him have unofficial naps throughout the day at this point.

For his night sleep, I will insert, in the example schedule, a six and a half hour stretch of sleep, although your baby may be sleeping more or less at night at this point. Just remember to start your cluster feeding routine about an hour and a half to two hours before wrapping him up and putting him down for the night, to make sure he is nice and full before his long stretch of sleep.

Here is the next example chart. It reflects these small changes to help you out:

Weeks 5 Through 7 Schedule

Line			
1	Use wake up time from 2 year chart	**9 AM**	Wake up for the day and Feed baby right away
2	Add 2 hours	**11 AM**	Feed Baby
3	Add half an hour	**11:30 AM**	Try to **keep baby awake** until official nap.
4	Add 1.5 hours	**1 PM**	Feed Baby until he falls asleep
5	Add half an hour	**1:30 PM**	**Official Nap Time!**
6	Add 3 hours	**4:30 PM**	Wake baby up from nap and feed right away
7	Add 2 hours	**6:30 PM**	Feed baby
8	Add 2 hours	**8:30 PM**	Feed baby
9	Add 2 hours	**10:30 PM**	Feed baby
10	Add 2 hours	**12:30 AM**	Feed Baby, try to **keep awake.** Start cluster feed.
11	Add 1 hour	**1:30 AM**	Start bedtime routine and feed baby again
12	Add half an hour	**2 AM**	Feed baby until he falls asleep for the night
13	Add half an hour	**2:30 AM**	**Official Sleep.** Say goodnight!
14	Add 6.5 hours	**9 AM**	Wake baby up for the day and feed.

Now here is a chart for you to fill out:

Weeks 5 Through 7 Schedule

Line			
Line 1	Use wake up time from 2 year chart		Wake up for the day and Feed baby right away
2	Add 2 hours		Feed Baby
3	Add half an hour		Try to **keep baby awake** until official nap.
4	Add 1.5 hours		Feed Baby until he falls asleep
5	Add half an hour		**Official Nap Time!**
6	Add 3 hours		Wake baby up from nap and feed right away
7	Add 2 hours		Feed baby
8	Add 2 hours		Feed baby
9	Add 2 hours		Feed baby
10	Add 2 hours		Feed Baby, try to **keep awake.** Start cluster feed.
11	Add 1 hour		Start bedtime routine and feed baby again
12	Add half an hour		Feed baby until he falls asleep for the night
13	Add half an hour		**Official Sleep.** Say goodnight!
14	Add 6.5 hours		Wake baby up for the day and feed.

Chapter 10

Week 8

*W*e have reached our goal time for eight consecutive hours of sleep! If your baby has not reached this goal yet, it's ok. Keep him on the five through seven week schedule until he has mastered that one (when he sleeps right through without waking for feedings and YOU have to wake him up at his wake up time rather than him waking up on his own before wake up time).

Don't graduate your baby to the next chart until he has aced the schedules in the current chart you are working with. The ages on the charts may be different for some babies, but the changes, from one chart to the next, reflect the natural progression and order you need to follow to have him sleep through the night.

At this point, he needs to stay awake two hours before his official naps and sleeps, and continue to start the cluster feeding approximately one and a half to two hours before bedtime. You can let him have unofficial naps throughout the day as long as you wake him two hours before the official sleeps. If you have trouble getting your baby to fall asleep for his official night sleeps, you should try to keep him awake for two and a half hours beforehand, rather than two hours.

Depending on your baby, he may not need as many as eight to 10 feedings per day, but can probably thrive on seven to eight feedings in a 24-hour period.

Somewhere around the eight-week mark, your baby may suddenly sleep much longer than you expected. If you've been struggling to even keep your baby on the newborn schedule with a five-hour stretch of sleep before his wake up time, sometimes they just suddenly get it over night and next thing you know they are sleeping eight straight hours, which can make parents worry! It's ok, this is normal! If this doesn't happen for you, don't worry, he should still get it slowly with the 30-minute increments method.

If your baby is doing incredibly well with the charts, move him up to the next chart. You don't have to wait until the age on the chart. The most important thing is that you are getting as much sleep as you can.

The next chart, for eight consecutive hours of sleep, will look like this, with only minor changes, from the five through seven week schedule, after line 10:

Week 8 Schedule

Line			
1	Use wake up time from 2 year chart	**9 AM**	Wake up for the day and Feed baby right away
2	Add 2 hours	**11 AM**	Feed Baby
3	Add half an hour	**11:30 AM**	Try to **keep baby awake** until official nap.
4	Add 1.5 hours	**1 PM**	Feed Baby until he falls asleep
5	Add half an hour	**1:30 PM**	**Official Nap Time!**
6	Add 3 hours	**4:30 PM**	Wake baby up from nap and feed right away
7	Add 2 hours	**6:30 PM**	Feed baby
8	Add 2 hours	**8:30 PM**	Feed baby
9	Add 2 hours	**10:30 PM**	Feed baby
10	Add half an hour	**11 PM**	Try to **keep baby awake.**
11	Add half an hour	**11:30 PM**	Start bedtime routine and cluster feed routine
12	Add 1 hour	**12:30 AM**	Feed baby until he falls asleep for the night.
13	Add half an hour	**1 AM**	**Official Sleep.** Say goodnight!
14	Add 8 hours	**9 AM**	Wake baby up for the day and feed.

Now here is your chart to fill out for reference:

Week 8 Schedule			
Line 1	Use wake up time from 2 year chart		Wake up for the day and Feed baby right away
2	Add 2 hours		Feed Baby
3	Add half an hour		Try to **keep baby awake** until official nap.
4	Add 1.5 hours		Feed Baby until he falls asleep
5	Add half an hour		**Official Nap Time!**
6	Add 3 hours		Wake baby up from nap and feed right away
7	Add 2 hours		Feed baby
8	Add 2 hours		Feed baby
9	Add 2 hours		Feed baby
10	Add half an hour		Try to **keep baby awake.**
11	Add half an hour		Start bedtime routine and cluster feed routine
12	Add 1 hour		Feed baby until he falls asleep for the night.
13	Add half an hour		**Official Sleep.** Say goodnight!
14	Add 8 hours		Wake baby up for the day and feed.

Chapter 11

Week 10

*N*ow that your baby is no longer newborn (I know, they grow too fast!), he is probably not as sleepy all the time, all day long. He will soon fall into needing just three nap times during the day. These nap times need to be structured even though two of the naps are unofficial naps, where you can let them fall asleep anywhere, and one is the official nap that you are used to, where he is wrapped up like a burrito and placed in his bassinet or crib.

Our goal, at this age, is to have your baby sleep 10 consecutive hours at night. Don't forget, if this is not happening yet, don't move on to the next chart until he masters the last one.

The two unofficial naps, we will be adding to this chart, are short naps. **Do your best to always keep your baby awake at this point if it is not time for an official or unofficial nap.**

Please note that **the official nap is changed to two and a half hours** now, to help encourage a longer night sleep.

The 10-week chart with three naps, and 10 hours of night sleep will look like this:

Week 10 Schedule

Line			
1	Use wake up time from 2 year chart	9 AM	Wake up for the day and Feed baby right away
2	Add 2 hours	11 AM	Feed Baby and **let sleep for 20 minutes** only.
3	Add half an hour	11:30 AM	Try to **keep baby awake** until official nap.
4	Add 1.5 hours	1 PM	Feed Baby until he falls asleep
5	Add half an hour	1:30 PM	**Official Nap Time!**
6	**Add 2.5 hours**	4 PM	Wake baby up from nap and feed.
7	Add 2 hours	6 PM	Feed baby.
8	Add 1 hour	7 PM	**Unofficial nap for 1 hour only.**
9	Add 1 hour	8 PM	Wake and feed baby.
10	Add 1.5 hours	9:30 PM	Start bedtime routine and cluster feed routine.
11	Add 1 hour	10:30 PM	Feed baby until he falls asleep for the night.
12	Add half an hour	11 PM	**Official Sleep.** Say goodnight!
13	Add 10 hours	9 AM	Wake baby up for the day and feed.

Here is your chart to fill out:

Week 10 Schedule

Line			
Line 1	Use wake up time from 2 year chart		Wake up for the day and Feed baby right away
2	Add 2 hours		Feed Baby and **let sleep for 20 minutes** only.
3	Add half an hour		Try to **keep baby awake** until official nap.
4	Add 1.5 hours		Feed Baby until he falls asleep
5	Add half an hour		**Official Nap Time!**
6	**Add 2.5 hours**		Wake baby up from nap and feed.
7	Add 2 hours		Feed baby.
8	Add 1 hour		**Unofficial nap for 1 hour only.**
9	Add 1 hour		Wake and feed baby.
10	Add 1.5 hours		Start bedtime routine and cluster feed routine.
11	Add 1 hour		Feed baby until he falls asleep for the night.
12	Add half an hour		**Official Sleep.** Say goodnight!
13	Add 10 hours		Wake baby up for the day and feed.

If your baby is not tired enough to go to bed for his official night sleeps at the time you entered in line 12 of your own chart,

94

reduce the nap from line 8 to half an hour, rather than one full hour. Try to make sure that your baby is awake for two hours before his official nap time from line 5, but now three hours before his official sleep in line 12.

It is more important to stick to the time block spacing rather than the actual time on the clock. If your baby falls asleep at the "wrong time," count the number of hours until the next sleep rather than trying to catch up with the clock. For example, if your baby "accidentally" sleeps his third nap from 8 p.m. – 9 p.m. rather than 7 p.m. – 8 p.m., he may not be tired enough to go to bed at 11 p.m., but will probably go to sleep by 12 a.m. Instead, take cues from your baby, and aim for that three-hour spacing, from the third nap to his official sleep time; then aim to follow the clock time the following day.

I've heard so many times people say to me, "What do I do? My baby just won't fall asleep tonight!" The first thing I ask is, "When was the last time he fell asleep, and for how long?" Then they might say, "We were visiting friends this evening, and he fell asleep in the car on the way home, for an hour from 9 p.m. – 10 p.m. We wanted to make it home for his 11 p.m. bedtime, but now he won't sleep, even though he falls asleep every night by 11 p.m.!"

My recommendation in cases like these is, it would be better to make sure that the baby has his three-hour awake stretch before putting him to bed for the night. Yes, unfortunately, he might not fall back to sleep until 1 a.m. if he woke up from a one-hour nap at 10 p.m., but it is better to do that than to get frustrated that you keep trying to put him to bed and it's not working because he's not tired enough.

Even if he falls asleep, the chances of him night waking are much higher than if you just wait for that three-hour stretch. If you do wait, the chances are he won't wake throughout the night, if he wasn't waking before, and it will be easier on you to sleep right through, than to have your baby wake through the night again.

Chapter 12

Week 12

*I*f your baby has responded well to the schedule thus far, he should be sleeping 12 consecutive hours now! If he isn't quite there yet, don't get discouraged; he will soon. Just keep his routine as similar as possible every day. If it is working well and if he is sleeping 12 straight hours, you will need to drop the first unofficial nap. In this case, the official nap will need to be moved earlier, because if he's used to dozing after being awake only two hours in the mornings, it will be too long for him to wait for the current time of the official nap. It is also a good idea at this point to shorten the third nap to 30 minutes, if you haven't already; and I trust that you have been shifting your baby's schedule to go to sleep earlier by 30 minutes, whenever he sleeps right through to his wake up time.

Once he has mastered sleeping 12 hours consecutively, you can try to feed him until he is ALMOST fully asleep, instead of fully asleep so he can start to learn to fall asleep on his own. (Learning this trick early will go a long way when he is a toddler!) A baby who is constantly rocked, to fall asleep, will eventually have trouble falling asleep unless he is rocked.

While it may seem like a great idea to do this, someday you may have another baby who is crying for your attention, but your toddler wants you to stay with him until he falls fully asleep. It can get stressful.

I am all for tender moments rocking your baby to sleep, but I recommend saving the rocking for the two unofficial naps, but not the two official sleeps. This way, he will learn to fall asleep when he is wrapped up as well as being rocked; so he has two options for successful sleep.

If you very gradually put your baby to bed, while he is less and less asleep, hopefully by age one, you will be able to put him in his crib fully awake, and have him still fall asleep because he knows it is time for bed. If you start to put him down, just before he is fully asleep, but it doesn't work as well as before, go back to putting him down when he is fully asleep, and revisit this method in two to four weeks.

I do not agree with the "cry it out" method. I feel it is unnecessary, especially when a solid routine has been laid out from the beginning. Three of my children never once went to sleep crying. My fourth is a little more vocal and sometimes she will cry when I leave the room; but I wait by her door and it turns out she is just re-adjusting in her "burrito wrap," or calling out to me to check if it is really bed time. Then she is quiet within a few minutes, and sleeps her 12 to 13 hours. There is no need to leave a baby crying until they are so exhausted and defeated that they eventually fall asleep from loneliness and fear. Can you imagine what that must feel like to someone so little when this big old world is still so new to them?

If you follow this routine, follow your instincts, and follow your baby's cues, he could fall asleep for the night and never feel like he needs to cry for more than two to three minutes.

Here is an example of what your baby could be doing by week 12, with a 12-hour night sleep; the first nap dropped altogether, the official nap moved earlier, and the third nap shortened to 30 minutes:

Week 12 Schedule

Line			
1	Use wake up time from 2 year chart	9 AM	Wake up for the day and Feed baby right away
2	Add 2 hours	11 AM	Feed Baby.
3	Add 1.5 hours	12:30 PM	**Feed baby until sleep. New Official Nap Time!**
4	Add 2.5 hours	3 PM	Wake baby up from nap and feed.
5	Add 2.5 hours	5:30 PM	Feed baby. **Let him nap 30 minutes only**
6	Add half an hour	6 PM	Keep him awake until bedtime
7	Add 1.5 hours	7:30 PM	Start bedtime routine and cluster feed routine.
8	Add 1 hour	8:30 PM	Feed baby until he falls asleep for the night.
9	Add half an hour	9 PM	**Official Sleep.** Say goodnight!
10	Add 12 hours	9 AM	Wake baby up for the day and feed.

Now here is your chart to fill out:

Week 12 Schedule

Line	Use wake up time from 2 year chart		
1	Use wake up time from 2 year chart		Wake up for the day and Feed baby right away
2	Add 2 hours		Feed Baby.
3	Add 1.5 hours		**Feed baby until sleep. New Official Nap Time!**
4	Add 2.5 hours		Wake baby up from nap and feed.
5	Add 2.5 hours		Feed baby. **Let him nap 30 minutes only**
6	Add half an hour		Keep him awake until bedtime
7	Add 1.5 hours		Start bedtime routine and cluster feed routine.
8	Add 1 hour		Feed baby until he falls asleep for the night.
9	Add half an hour		**Official Sleep.** Say goodnight!
10	Add 12 hours		Wake baby up for the day and feed.

Chapter 13

The Next Stage

*B*ecause babies can be so different, from one to the next, it is very difficult to predict his next stage, by his age. He could be following the schedule we introduced to him in week 12, for several months.

In the next stage, we will be dropping the last nap, and moving the official nap back to the original time, one hour later. DO NOT skip the official nap! Believe it or not, he should be able to have this nap until he goes to school. I had my first son still napping during the summer months until he was six years old.

How do you judge whether your baby is ready for the changes in the next step or not?

1. Take cues from your baby. The 12-week schedule has a three and a half hour gap from wake up time to the official nap time. If you are finding that your baby is still wide awake after this amount of time, it is time to try pushing his official nap forward, making the gap between four, and four and a half hours of awake time before you put him down to sleep.

2. If your baby is not tired enough to go to bed on time at night, it may be time to drop the last nap altogether.

3. If your baby was sleeping very well at night, but now he seems to have changed and he is starting to wake up, that could also be a sign that he needs to drop the last nap.

If your baby is giving you these signs before you start him on solid foods, your new schedule will look like this:

Months 4 To 6 Schedule
(IF baby is ready. If not, stick with 12 week schedule)

Line 1	Use wake up time from 2 year chart	9 AM	Wake up for the day and Feed baby right away
2	Add 2 hours	11 AM	Feed Baby.
3	Add 2 hours	1 PM	**Feed baby until he falls sleep.**
4	Add half an hour hours	1:30 PM	**New Official Nap Time!**
5	Add 2.5 hours	4 PM	Wake baby up from nap and feed.
6	Add 2 hours	6 PM	Feed and Keep him awake until bedtime
7	Add 1.5 hours	7:30 PM	Start bedtime routine and cluster feed routine.
8	Add 1 hour	8:30 PM	Feed baby until he falls asleep for the night.
9	Add half an hour	9 PM	**Official Sleep.** Say goodnight!
10	Add 12 hours	9 AM	Wake baby up for the day and feed.

Keep in mind, it is possible that he will not be ready for this chart until after his first birthday! You be the judge, but either way, this is what your baby's schedule should change to when he needs the change.

Now here is your schedule to fill out:

Months 4 To 6 Schedule
(IF baby is ready. If not, stick with 12 week schedule)

Line	Use wake up time		Wake up for the day and
1	from 2 year chart		Feed baby right away
2	Add 2 hours		Feed Baby.
3	Add 2 hours		**Feed baby until he falls sleep.**
4	Add half an hour hours		**New Official Nap Time!**
5	Add 2.5 hours		Wake baby up from nap and feed.
6	Add 2 hours		Feed and Keep him awake until bedtime
7	Add 1.5 hours		Start bedtime routine and cluster feed routine.
8	Add 1 hour		Feed baby until he falls asleep for the night.
9	Add half an hour		**Official Sleep.** Say goodnight!
10	Add 12 hours		Wake baby up for the day and feed.

Notice how the actual sleeping times are now almost identical to your 2-year-old chart. The only difference is that the official sleep is still two and a half hours here, instead of two hours.

110

Once your baby is following this routine, he may continue this way for a couple of years. If you find that your baby doesn't seem tired enough to go to bed on time, I would suggest you cut the official nap to two hours so that there is a five and a half hour wake time gap before his night sleep. Once this happens, the sleep times will be identical to your two-year-old chart.

Your baby may need his official nap shortened to two hours at approximately age 18 months to 30 months. If you choose to shorten the official nap, shorten it by waking him from his nap earlier, rather than putting him down for his nap later. For example, always keep the time gap from wake up time to official nap time four and a half hours. To shorten the nap, make the gap between the official nap to his official sleep, six hours, instead of five, or five and a half hours. This will help make sure he is tired enough for his 12 hour sleep at night.

Don't forget; the next stage schedule happens at many different ages for different babies. Your baby may get here at four months old, but that is rare. My main objective, with this sleep schedule, is to have your baby sleeping eight hours by eight weeks, and 12 hours by 12 weeks. If you are sleeping at night, you are succeeding no matter what age your child needs to drop all the naps!

When you decide to start feeding your baby solid foods, the only difference it will make to the charts is that he probably will not need to cluster feed with his milk, so early before bed. You can start the cluster feeding about an hour before putting him to bed, rather than one and a half to two hours before bed.

By now, I'm sure you know your baby so well that you have a good grasp on his cues and routines; and you can adjust things as you see fit. The main goal is to have a four and a half hour wake time gap between wake up time and official nap time, and a five and a half to six hour gap, from when he wakes up from his nap, until he goes to bed for the night.

Chapter 14

Starting Solids, Supplementing, And Growth Spurts

*Y*ou can start solid foods when you feel it's necessary, however, doctors recommend starting solids around six months of age. If you are nursing and you want to ensure an abundant milk supply, I suggest that you nurse right before feeding the solids at each meal, so that your baby is still drinking a full portion of milk.

Although feeding your baby solid foods can help him sleep longer at night, your baby absolutely CAN still sleep a full 12 hours, without waking, on just your breast milk alone. You do not need to supplement earlier than six months with formula or solids if you are producing enough milk.

If your baby sometimes gets very fussy and cries a lot when you try to nurse him, it is very common for a mother's first thought to be "maybe he's not getting enough milk?"

If breastfeeding is important to you, and you want to continue nursing for quite some time, consider other possible issues before deciding to supplement before the six-month mark, because supplementing will decrease your milk production.

1. If your baby seems very hungry, but angry, and even hits your chest when he tries to eat, and you feel like your tanks are running on empty, it is possible that he is having a growth spurt. Growth spurts can be a very difficult time for any mom.

Your baby may seem upset and demanding and he will act like you stopped producing breast milk, but what is in fact happening is he is signaling to your body to produce more milk to meet his growing little body. Not only will his growth spurt increase your milk volume, but the actual milk changes to meet his new nutritional needs! I find this so amazing.

This may happen for up to three days, where you feel like all you are doing is nursing your baby; and the crying can be very wearing on you and difficult to handle, but once he has increased your milk production from his suckling, he will want to sleep a lot for two to three days.

Understanding this process can help you get through it because you won't be wondering if you are doing something wrong and why your baby is so upset no matter what you do. Keep it up and things will return to normal soon!

It can be tricky to stick to his sleep schedule during a growth spurt. If you are having difficulty with keeping him on track during a growth spurt, I would suggest you back track by one chart. For example, if he has already dropped his last nap, go back to the chart that lets him have a nap so it can be well timed out for his night sleep. If he starts napping all over the place, it will affect his night sleep. Once the growth spurt is over (about five days) and he returns to the baby you once knew, he should be able to resume his regular schedule fairly easily after that.

2: If your baby cries a lot at the breast, seems mad at you and even bites you, it is possible that the problem is that he is teething, not that you are not producing enough milk.

3: If your baby is clenching his fists and seems to flex every muscle in his body while screaming at you when trying to nurse and trying to make you feel like you are doing absolutely everything wrong, it is possible that either he has indigestion, or that he is over stimulated and he got too tired earlier than usual. Did you run a lot of errands today? Were you in a noisy environment for a while with him? Did he miss a nap?

These are different possibilities that you can consider, when his fussiness makes you think you don't have enough milk for him. Always use your instincts, if you think there is a problem with your production, ask a health care professional for advice. But you still can train a child to sleep properly, and all night, with breast milk alone.

So how do you fit feeding solids into the sleep schedules? Well, only you will know which chart your baby is currently following at his age, and it also depends which month you start him on solids, so I cannot give you exact times in this case. My general tips, however, would be to pick one of the scheduled milk feeding sessions, give your baby the milk as usual first, then do the solids right after.

Pick a daytime scheduled milk feeding though, to start. You probably want to give your baby solids soon before bed thinking it may be better for his sleep, but the reason I suggest daytime feedings, at the beginning, is so that you will be awake to check for any possible allergic reactions your baby may have to the new foods.

After a couple of weeks, if your baby is not having any adverse reactions to anything he has tried, by all means, feed him in the late evening if you wish. Just remember, if you are nursing, do the milk right before the solid meal to help sustain your milk production.

Chapter 15

Where should my baby sleep?

*Y*our baby can sleep wherever you want him to sleep; but if it were me, I know I wouldn't be able to sleep soundly if I had a baby in my bed waking me up with every little cute noise they make, every time they stir (which isn't always so cute at 4 a.m.!) Plus, every time he opens his eyes and sees you, he will decide he needs you for something.

It's actually part of my sleep method NOT to co-sleep. If you teach your baby to sleep on their own, right from the beginning, you won't have as many transitions for them to get used to later on, you will sleep more soundly earlier on, and chances are, he will sleep longer.

If your baby has been sleeping with you, in your bed, for six months, it will be hard for him to learn to sleep on his own, once you decide you want your bed to yourself again. *"Mommy has always been there, and suddenly she's not? Ahhh!"*

Every time they make a change, it can affect their sleep, which will affect your sleep. I know how precious it is to sleep next to your baby. That's why the unofficial naps, at the beginning, allow for a lot of freedom. They allow you to nap with your baby early on, but for the future of your own sleep, (and intimacy with your spouse), having their official naps and sleeps, in their own bassinet and crib, will go a long way for your own personal sleep quality…and theirs.

I do suggest having them sleep, in a bassinet or crib in your room, for the first three to four weeks. If you are nursing, and your baby is only a few feet from you, your body and your milk will send you a signal just before your baby wakes up, to wake you up because your baby wants to feed. This may not happen for everyone, but it does happen a lot. So if they do wake up for a feeding, while you are sleeping, the baby is right there for you to nurse, then make sure he is still wrapped and put him right back down in his bassinet or crib.

The reason I am suggesting, to only keep him in your room for the first few weeks, is because babies stir often in their sleep, but most times they fall back into a deep sleep on their own without needing a feeding if they are not disturbed.

If you wake up every time your baby stirs, and you pick him up thinking he is hungry or needs you for something, at times that he would have otherwise fallen back asleep on his own, you will not get the best quality sleep that you can get, and your baby will not learn to work little things out on his own. They may let out a cry when they pass gas or try to stretch into a different position and then a lot of times they fall back asleep.

Following the schedules is very important, because the charts can help teach you how long your baby could be sleeping without milk at certain ages; so if they cry for a minute or two, you will know that they may fall back to sleep; or you can try putting a soother in his mouth to lull him back to sleep if it is within the time frame that he likely doesn't need milk.

If you have followed the schedule closely, and he has had all the feedings he needs, before that five-hour stretch of sleep as a newborn, chances are, he's not waking for another feed. If you teach him when he is getting milk and when he is not, he will fall into the sleeping habit at night much sooner.

Of course, use your instincts on this as well! Don't leave him crying for more than a few minutes, if the soother didn't work and he didn't fall back asleep. He may need milk if he is having a growth spurt or if he didn't feed long enough before bed. It could also be that he needs a diaper change. If you let him get too upset, it will be much harder to get him to go back to sleep.

Don't forget to avoid changing his diaper during his official sleep hours unless it is dirty or very wet. The less you disturb his sleep and his burrito swaddle, the easier he will fall back to sleep.

Once you move him into his own room, at around three to four weeks old, you will be able to sleep through his little grunting noises just fine, and he will more likely be able to learn to work out his own small issues. Having a baby monitor is ideal because if he does wake for milk, while you are still working on mastering the schedules, you will still hear him and you can get to him before he gets too upset.

If he started off in a bassinet, and you want to put him in the crib, start by placing the actual bassinet IN the crib if possible. He will already be familiar with the feeling of his bed while getting used to the new environment. The more gradual the changes you give him are, the more likely you will have success, and I also believe very minor gradual changes can help prevent them from suffering with anxiety and night terrors.

If he is in a bassinet inside the crib for a while, and is quite used to that now, when you take the bassinet away, consider putting the bassinet's padding and the same bedding in the crib with him. He will be familiar with some things, while changing others, which will also help him transition well.

Chapter 16

How To Teach Your Baby
To Wake Up Happy.

*D*on't you love hearing stories mothers tell about how their baby sleeps all night, then wakes up without even crying and lets her sleep in, while he plays alone in his crib until she goes to get him?

You might think that this scenario, in your own household, would take place, only in your dreams. Some babies just have a peaceful temperament, and waking up happy, and being able to occupy himself so you can sleep longer, may come naturally to him. Many babies however, will need to be taught and guided into allowing you this luxury. I would like to share my ideas with you on things you can try to help teach your baby to wake up without crying or wailing for you, as if it's some kind of daily emergency.

I like to start everything with newborns, because we don't have to worry about back tracking to correct the behavior, or to teach them something brand new, when they have been doing it one way their whole lives. It's never too early to start. But starting later can work as well!

Starting from newborn, I believe that it is important, for the first while (a couple of months) to do your best to make sure your baby is fully asleep, when you put him down; and do your best to be the one to wake him before he wakes up on his own. This will help your baby associate his bed with positive feelings because let's face it, sleep is great! When you wake him, talk to your baby for five minutes before taking him out of his bed.

Speak with a wonderfully comforting, happy voice tone and give lots of smiles, rub his head, stroke his cheeks, etc.

Believe it or not, even as young as your baby is, he will associate all this with happy feelings, while still lying down in his crib. If your baby tends to seem very hungry, when he wakes up at this stage, make sure you don't use this morning routine for more than five minutes, or he may get frustrated. If he starts to cry, and you know it's just a "pick me up" cry and not an "I'm hungry cry," try to distract him with different facial expressions, or new happy sentences. You can also try to dangle a new toy for him to look at; anything that will distract him so he can calm down. Once he calms down, you can pick him up afterwards.

Having you there when he wakes up in his crib will help him to not feel like he has to get out of his crib the moment he wakes up.

From about six months of age, (could be different timing for different babies) hopefully you are able to put your baby down to sleep, before he is fully asleep so he can fall asleep on his own. You can also let your baby wake up on his own for a few minutes.

If you hear him awake in his room, but he is not crying, don't go in just yet. Wait five minutes and then go in. Don't wait until your baby is crying for you to go in, if you can help it. I understand, many times you may not be able to catch him before he cries, but when you can, it's good to do so. If the only time you get to him is when you hear him cry, he will believe, and learn, surprisingly quickly, that he HAS to cry to have you come to get him.

If you go in after five minutes, before he cries when he wakes up, he will soon realize you are coming to get him no matter what, and he doesn't have to use his cry as a signal to get your attention.

If you are having trouble and you can't get him to be alone for five minutes without crying, back track to trying to wake him up before he wakes up on his own, and chat with him for a while before you pick him up.

Unfortunately this means you may have to set your alarm earlier, but then you can try the five minute method again in a couple of weeks.

Babies waking up happy will also depend on how many consecutive hours of sleep they got that night. If they have succeeded in sleeping through the night. The longer they sleep, the happier they will be, and the hunger pangs will also not be as strong if they have slept well.

Once you are able to master this five-minute trick, and he is able to wait five minutes for you to come in the room, (possibly around age six to nine months), start putting a few toys at the foot of his crib so he will see them when he moves around in the morning; but they won't be near his head to distract him from sleeping through the night. Make sure the toys are large enough that he can't put them in his mouth and choke, and also avoid toys with long strings attached to them. If you are able to hear him wake in the morning, and it seems he has found the treasures you put in his crib to peak his interest, start extending the five-minute method to between seven and 10 minutes. But again, go in BEFORE he cries, to greet him, if possible.

Try switching the toys up, every few nights, so he has something new and interesting to discover, that he can think about before deciding that he needs you. Slowly and very gradually extend the time before entering your baby's room. When he is happy with 10 minutes alone, go to 12 or 15 minutes, and go in before he cries. Don't extend the times until he is doing really well with the current time frame.

Babies don't just automatically understand this stuff. You have to take the time to teach him that waking up is nothing to cry about. All your actions and routines will give your baby an idea what he can expect from you, and what he has to do or doesn't have to do to get your attention.

I will cover suggestions on how to get your toddler to let you sleep longer, in the next chapter.

Chapter 17

Switching Your Child To A Toddler Bed
(And Keeping Him In It At Night).

*M*ost of the time, under normal circumstances, the decision on when to switch your baby to a toddler bed is based on personal preference. I actually think the older, the better! I'm not talking about age 10 here, but if you switch your baby too early; before he is able to understand that he should stay in his room at night, guess what? The chances are much higher that you may end up having a nightly visitor in your room, waking you from every dream that you missed out on, from when he was first born. The older they are, when they switch, the better they will understand when you explain to them that you need to have a full night's sleep so you will have enough energy to play with him during the day. (They will understand more, if you relate your sleep to something that affects them).

My suggestion would be to not even worry about switching them into a toddler bed until they are daytime potty trained. You won't want them stuck in their crib so they can't use the potty. (Or trying to climb out of their crib to use the potty). That would just reverse your potty training efforts.

Potty training success can be anywhere from age two to age three and a half, on average. Once you feel that your child is interested enough in trying to use a potty at night on his own, this is a good time to switch their bed. You can actually tell them that it's a special present for them as a reward for doing so well on the potty. When they feel like it was a special reward gift for something wonderful they have done, they will like bedtime that much more.

Next, when you have switched their bed, make sure you remind them every night for a while: "Ok sweetie, now stay in your room until I come to get you in the morning. Mommy and daddy need to sleep too." It helps to put a special night potty in their room so that they are not roaming the hallways at night, because that will also give them the idea to come into your room to wake you, since they're already walking around.

Make a big deal out of the night potty in their room, while adding reminders in your sentences that they need to stay in their room at night. For example: "Wow it would be so exciting to see if you used your potty when I come and wake you in the morning! That would be a great surprise for mommy after I wake up!"

If you have just found my book, and your baby is already a toddler, who already comes out of their room and wakes you, for no good reason, and he has had this habit for a while and you don't know how to reverse it, I really feel for you! Start by explaining that you need to sleep and you would be so proud of him if he could be a big boy and stay in his room at night for mommy and daddy. Make sure you explain this to your toddler during the daytime when you know he is paying attention. If he still comes out of his room to wake you without a valid reason, consider setting up a reward chart system.

A suggestion for this is: you could hang a calendar on the back of his door so he will see it before he leaves his room in the middle of the night, hopefully reminding him to reconsider waking you. You can tell him that he will earn a sticker for every night that he does not wake you or come out of his room. A certain amount of stickers earned, in a specific time period, will translate into a privilege. For example: Extra TV time, a video game, a toy from the dollar store…pick something that he wouldn't normally get, so it can be a greater motivator for him, to stay in his room at night.

The older he is, the harder he has to work for it. So to start off, especially if he is younger, let's say you offer him an extra privilege for every five stickers he can earn in a 10-day period. As time goes on, you can raise the stakes until his night roaming has stopped completely. So now maybe he has to earn seven or eight stickers in a 10-day period to earn his privilege. Whatever you introduce and however your introduce it, it is important to STICK TO IT for it to work best.

If your toddler stays in his room at night, but your biggest nightmare is him waking you at the crack of dawn, when you didn't need to wake up for another hour, remember to remind him before bed time, to stay in his room, in the morning, until you come to get him (within reason of course). Tell him he can look at some picture books, or play with some toys in his room.

If your sleep is as important to you as mine is to me, you must try to think one step ahead of him. They will try anything to convince you that it's a good idea to wake you up when you don't want to be woken up yet. If he says: "But mommy, I'm too hungry!" Consider putting a small snack of cheerios (or something that won't dirty your carpets or walls) next to his bed every night so he can munch on them when he gets up in the morning.

If he says "I'm too bored without you!" Give him rotating ideas before bedtime on what he can do in the morning, if he wakes up before you. For example, give him paper and crayons (unless he tends to use the walls as his canvas) and say "can you color a special picture for me and show it to me after I wake up, to surprise me?" If he says: "But I just miss you!" Reply with "I'll be with you all day long, and if I get enough sleep, I will be much happier!"

As soon as you give in once, and don't correct him when he wakes you, when you don't want him to, he will start to find reasons to do it again and again. Give him an inch and he will take a mile. You can give him all the love he needs when it is an appropriate time to be awake. Don't forget to not reward him with conversation if he gets up at night. Walk him back to his room without talking. The only word you should use during night waking for a toddler is: "bedtime". That's it. No other words. Don't even say: "tell me in the morning." He will eventually get bored of this when he realizes he won't be getting any reaction or conversation out of you. He will stop getting up if it's all for nothing. Just silently walk him to his room and explain, in the morning, why you weren't talking to him.

Another tip is to avoid doing time outs in his bedroom as a form of discipline. This will cause him to associate his bedroom with negative feelings, and be less likely to want to camp out in there alone for the night. Instead, you can do your time outs facing a corner, sitting on the stairs, or something he will find very boring. It is best to keep his feelings about his bedroom safe, and that he will see it as a happy place. Then he will more likely want to stay in there at night, to sleep.

Chapter 18

Frequently Asked Questions

*H*ere is a short list of some of the common questions I get asked from tired parents, and some suggested answers, that will hopefully help you.

Question #1: *I just found your book, but my baby is 12 months old and not sleeping through the night. How do I incorporate your schedule when I didn't start it from the newborn stage?*

Answer: Although it is easier to start incorporating my sleep method right from day one, there's no reason you can't have success when starting it late.

Try logging your baby's sleep and nap habits for a few days and compare your notes to see which chart schedule your baby's habits most closely resemble. Even if your baby is 12 months old, he may match the four-month chart with his habits. The ages on the charts are based on the ages that your child is able to attain these goals if you start the method right from the beginning.

Although the progression of the charts is the natural path your baby's sleep habits should take, the age that they master each chart will be different depending on certain factors. Once you pinpoint which chart your baby's sleep habits compare the closest to, do your best to adjust things, as needed, to follow the time blocks specified in each chart so that his awake time gaps and sleep time gaps match the chart.

For example, if your baby is getting sleepy, but the chart says nap time isn't for another hour, do what you can to keep him awake until the right time (bath time, showing him a new toy, playing with him, anything you can think of to shift the nap to the proper time). Then try to put him down at the right time. Incorporating the lighting, music, white noise, and blocking out the sunlight are the easy parts.

My method works best when all components are incorporated together however, an older baby that hasn't been used to being wrapped like a burrito likely won't enjoy it like newborns do!

Hopefully, you will be able to get your older baby to follow the proper time block within two to three weeks. Then proceed with the instructions found in the chapter that has the chart your baby is now following which will give you tips on what they might start to do when they are ready to attempt the next chart.

Question #2 *Everything was going perfectly for a few months, and now my baby is waking up at night again. Why is this happening and what can I do?*

Answer: This is common! There are several reasons why this happens. If your baby started waking again at night, and it's been more than a few nights of this when he is NOT on the two-year-old chart, it may be a sign that he is ready to move onto the next chart.

Other reasons he may have trouble sleeping can be if he is teething, not feeling well, or having a growth spurt. Babies can also get too excited to sleep when they are ready to learn to do something new, or if they just learned something new.

A baby who is at the stage of rolling over, (around four or five months) may be too excited about the fact that he has accomplished this. I bet you have trouble sleeping when you are very excited about something too! Other exciting milestones that may trigger night waking again include:

-Sitting unassisted for the first time (five to six months)

-Pulling himself to a standing position (six to seven months)

-Cruising (walking while holding on to furniture)(seven to nine months)

-Walking unassisted (nine months to 15 months)

Then of course when they're between 15 and 18 months, they may start to get a little mischievous, and try things out on you to see what he can get away with. My suggestion for all of those things is to continue with all of your routines normally, as if nothing has changed! Once he realizes that you're not going to let him get up for the day at 4 a.m. to practice his new milestones (he will definitely try to test you, for a few days to a couple of weeks). If you stick to it and do everything exactly the same, he should eventually fall back into the pattern of the chart he was on.

Don't reward them with a change of routine or conversation, if it is the middle of the night. If you don't give him anything exciting to wake up to, hopefully he will be too bored to try to stay awake until morning when you get interesting to him again.

Question #3: *I thought I was doing well with my nursing schedule, but all of a sudden, all my baby wants to do is nurse, it seems like I don't have enough milk, and he won't go to sleep! What do I do?*

Answer: These are classic signs of growth spurts. Please refer to chapter 14 to read more about growth spurts and how to handle them. The chances are you do have enough milk, but you just need to keep at it until your baby increases your milk production to meet the new demands.

Question #4: *My baby just cries every time I take him off the breast and try to put him down to sleep. Is he getting enough milk?*

Answer: You will know if your baby is getting enough milk by tracking his wet diapers, the consistency of his bowel movements, and his weight gain. If you have concerns about your milk supply, please check with a health care professional.

Young babies like to suck, soothe and be held seemingly at all times. If you are quite sure he is getting enough milk, and that he is not having a growth spurt, it's possible that the issue is simply that your baby loves you so much he finds it hard to be away from you. It is important for you to teach him to settle, without you, so you can get some rest, or get things done, so in this case, I would suggest maybe giving him a soother, so he can soothe on his own, and using the "fake arms wrap" technique is a good trick to try as well. Trick him into feeling like he is being held.

You can stay with him in the room and tell him it's ok, and say soothing things until he falls asleep, so that he doesn't feel like he is alone trying to deal with his transition into the world. Unfortunately, holding him ALL the time, and not letting him attempt to work things out on his own (as long as he is not too upset) will only hinder both of you in the long run. I know it is hard, but it is well worth it!

Nothing happens automatically with babies! It's a long learning process for both you AND your baby. Everybody goes through it, but not everyone talks about it. You are not alone!

Question #5: *My baby always falls asleep at the "wrong time" when I am running errands. What can I do to stay on schedule?*

Answer: Most babies fall asleep with movement, especially in vehicles or long stroller rides. If your baby is a newborn, it doesn't matter much when he falls asleep throughout the day, as long as you stop to nurse him on schedule, and try to make sure you are home to keep him awake for half an hour before his official sleeps.

Let's say you are grocery shopping, and your baby starts to get sleepy and you know he will miss his next scheduled nap time if you let him fall asleep. I would suggest changing things up!

If your baby is older (six months and up), if he is sitting up in a shopping cart, he is less likely to fall asleep than if he is in a stroller. If he tends to stay awake when in a carrier, try that as well.

If he seems sleepy, no matter what you do, move him from stroller, to cart, to carrier, back to cart, back to stroller...keep stirring him so he will hopefully be ready for a peaceful nap at home where he will just be thankful that you're no longer bothering him. If he's just too cranky and starts crying in the store, because he is TOO tired, it's best to just give up the battle for the day and try again next time, or try to run your errands earlier so he is not so tired.

If it's at all possible, try to plan your activities around the schedules. If you know he gets drowsier in the afternoons, consider running your errands with him in the evenings, or vice versa.

If you are in the car and on the way home when he starts falling asleep, pass him an interesting toy, or start singing something upbeat, turn the interior lights off and on, open the windows...anything to keep him stirred until he can nap in his bed. Just keep your eyes on the road! You might feel like you're crazy or going overboard, but if it works and you succeed in getting him to sleep in his bed so you can take a nap, who cares! It is still better than him sleeping in the car for 15 minutes, then being cranky all evening because he didn't sleep long enough!

It's a lot of work and planning during the days, but if you are sleeping better at night than you would be if you weren't on top of all the planning, it is still easier than having to be awake at times when you're overly exhausted.

When you're exhausted, everything is so much harder than it should be, and the only way around it is to sleep; so all the extra planning is worth it!

Question #7: *My baby doesn't ever seem to want to nap more than 20 minutes when your schedule says she should be sleeping two and a half hours. How do I get him to sleep longer?*

Answer: Again, try to make sure you are following the time block spacing more closely than the actual clock time. If your baby is not sleeping long enough during his official nap time, it's most likely because he's not awake long enough before you put him down for a nap.

If the chart you are working with isn't working because you feel that your baby no longer needs as much sleep, it's time to skip ahead to the next chart. BUT it can also mean that he is OVERtired.

How can you tell the difference? When babies are overtired, they can seem really wired, like they can't stop moving. They may also be cranky, or too whiny for no other apparent reason, but they have trouble sleeping because they are just over stimulated.

In this case, I would rewind back one chart, and maybe he needs the unofficial nap again before the long stretch of sleep for the official nap.

If you feel like all the timings are right, and there's no other apparent reason why your baby does not want to sleep longer than 20 minutes, like no growth spurts, no major milestones achieved, no teething, etc, when your baby wakes up after 20 minutes, if he is not crying, see how long he will play in his bed. If he is crying for you, consider going into his room, don't say anything, (or if he is older, you can whisper "it's nap time" and say nothing else). Just try a soother to calm him, or fix his blanket so that you are sending him clues that you are there for him, but you are expecting him to sleep.

Do your best to keep him in his room during the time that you expect him to sleep; and stick to the routine every day, and hopefully he will finally figure out that this is the time he stays in the room, whether he is awake or not; and when you take him out of bed, is the time that it's ok to play. Don't just try for two days and give up. I would say stick to it for at least a month to see if he will eventually figure out the routine.

Keep in mind, it is practically impossible for them to figure out the routine if it is different every day; and then you won't even know when to expect that you can look forward to getting your rest, or when you can possibly even cook dinner or take a shower for that matter.

Often times, it might feel like things are just not working, but the key is the routine. Do the same thing every day, and he should figure it out based on their learned memories from previous days.

Question #8: *Now that my baby is 16 months old, she doesn't want to nap anymore. Should I skip the official nap because she's older now?*

Answer: This is a common age for the little ones to try new things on you again. If I were you, I would not skip the official nap until they go to school! If they do not need quite as much sleep anymore, you can shorten the nap, but don't skip it.

This is your break! It's your time to regroup, your time to relax. You might even need this more than your baby does! Plus, your baby will be happier if he gets some rest.

If he doesn't want to nap, tell him it's now called "quiet time," and put a few new toys or picture books in his crib that he can look at to keep his interest going, and you can also have some quiet time.

The thing is, if YOU want your child to nap, then you tell him it's nap time or quiet time. Don't let a toddler make household decisions for you. If, when they are two years old, they say: "I'm not even tired!" but you still want and need that quiet time, say "You don't have to fall asleep, just have some quiet time, look at a book, or play with your blocks in your bed and I will come and get you in an hour." Chances are, he will end up falling asleep anyways! They just like to fight naps when they still actually need them. I can't imagine why. I would never fight a nap now!

If it doesn't bother you to have them up with you for 12 hours a day and you don't need that break, and your child fights the nap and that's ok with you, by all means, let the nap go. Just make sure that the parents are the ones making the decisions and not the child.

Make sure you are taking care of yourself and meeting your own needs as well. Your child needs you to be strong to take care of him; so make sure you make decisions that will work for you, and stick to them! You are doing just fine.

~~~~~~~~~~~~~~~~~~~~~~~~~~~~~~~~~~~~~~~

If you have any questions that I have not covered here, or if you need or would like extra advice, please write to me directly at HeavenlySleep@hotmail.com, and I will do my best to help you.

If you live in the Durham region of Ontario, or the greater Toronto area, I offer one-on-one consultations, including sleep coaching and nursing advice. Please contact me for information and a fee schedule.

If you have any comments or testimonies on how my sleep method has worked for you, I would love to hear from you!

Sweet Dreams!

Prayer

I sincerely hope that you have found this book to be a blessing, and that it helps you get the sleep you need, to care for, and raise your beautiful baby.

If you don't know Jesus Christ as your personal Savior, and you feel you would like to know Him personally and have a daily relationship with Him, I would like to pray with you. God is no respecter of persons. What the Lord has done for me, He can also do for you:

Please pray this prayer with me:

Dear God,

I come to You in the name of Jesus. I admit that my heart is not right with You and that I am a sinner. I believe You died on the cross for me to save me from my sins. I don't want to live this life making decisions on my own anymore. I need You in my life. I don't want to just know about You, I want to know You personally. Please come into my heart and wash me clean from my sins by the blood of Jesus, so I can experience Your love and Your peace and so I can start a personal relationship with You. I want to make You Lord of my life, in Jesus' name,

AMEN!

May God bless you with your new walk with the Lord, and with your sleeping baby!